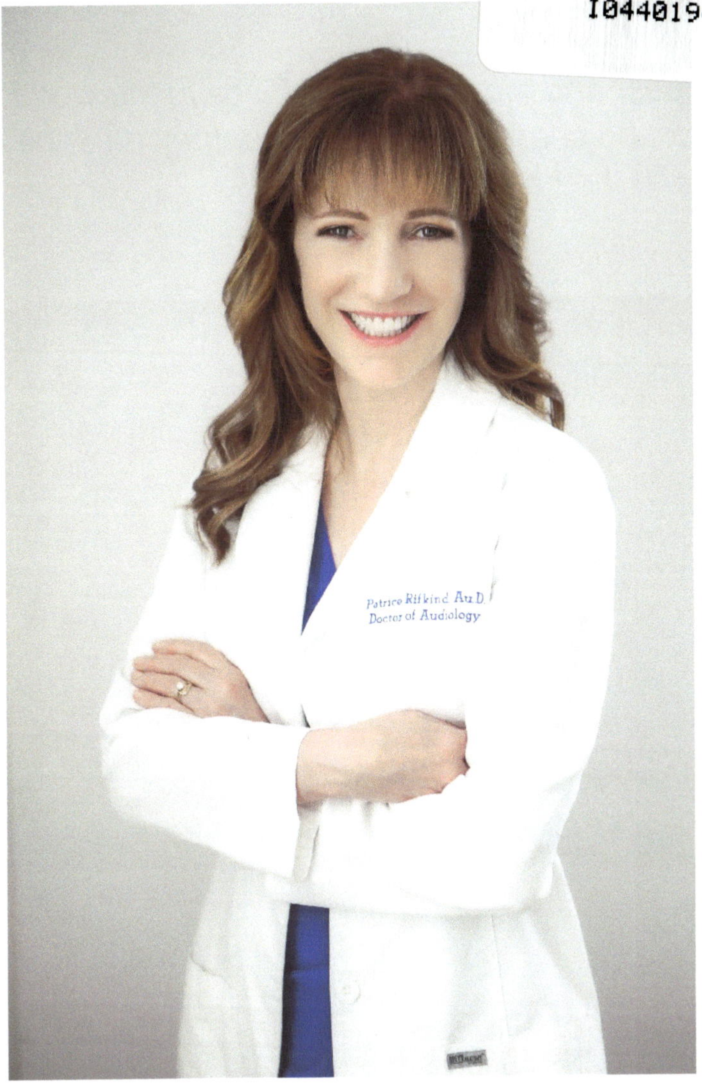

HEAR BETTER

A GUIDE TO FINDING THE BEST HEARING HEALTHCARE

by Patrice Rifkind, Au.D.

The best and most beautiful things in the world cannot be seen or even touched, they must be felt with the heart.

Helen Keller

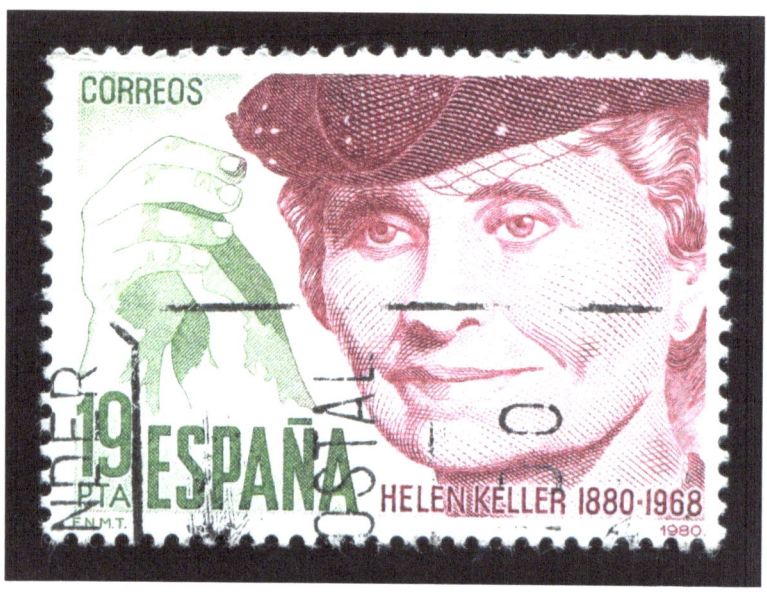

Table of Contents

ISBN: 978-1536987928

Introduction

by Cydney Fox, Au.D.

Dr. Patrice Rifkind, Au.D. was my competitor. We both had audiology practices in the Santa Clarita Valley of Los Angeles County and sought to help the same hearing impaired patients. We ended up at the same Health Fairs, Senior Citizen events, and citywide health symposiums. Everywhere I turned, she was there with her charming smile and amazing level of enthusiasm.

She turned up at all the events sponsored by hearing aid companies to teach us about their products. She showed up at all the Continuing Educational Units that I attended both state wide and nationally. I finally decided to get to know her.

It was to my benefit. She is a knowledgeable person who loves working with hearing aids and helping those with hearing problems. She cannot learn enough about hearing aids and how she can use them to make someone's life better. Nothing makes her happier than a patient who can HEAR all the sweet notes of a full life.

When I decided to stop dispensing hearing aids, I needed to refer all my patients to someone who I knew would take good care of them. I immediately sent all Patrice's contact information. When my husband needed new hearing aids, I sent him to Patrice and I didn't feel the need to accompany him to his appointments. I knew he would get what he needed. When I need some kind of touch up on my hearing aids, I schedule an appointment with Patrice. She really is my "go to" person when I have questions or want to bounce ideas off her. I guess you can say Dr. Patrice Rifkind is the *"audiologist's audiologist."*

I value her point of view. I value her commitment to the profession. I value her dedication to her patients. And I am proud that she asked me to write this introduction for her book.

Cydney Fox, Au.D.

Doctor of Audiology
Board Certified, Audiology
Former member of the California Speech Pathology/Audiology Licensing Board
Past president of the California Academy of Audiology

1 – STEP INTO MY OFFICE

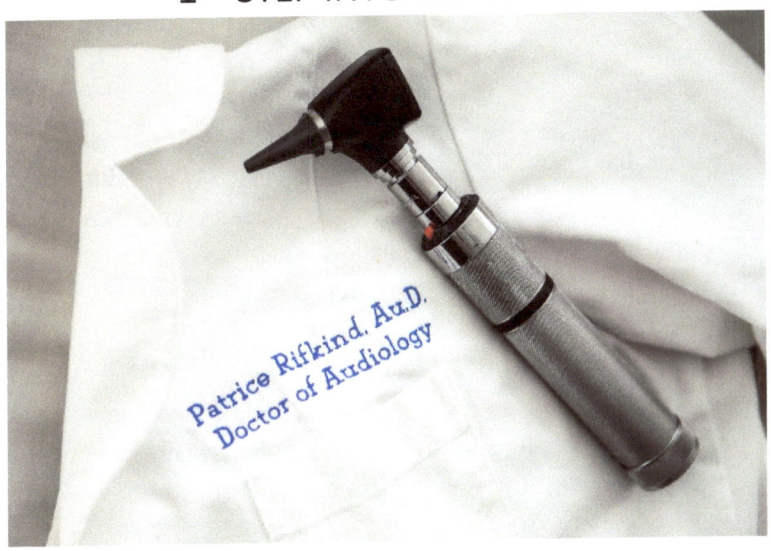

Welcome to my office. I suspect you are here because you or someone you know is dealing with a hearing issue. You've come to the right place. I am an audiologist, a hearing specialist with a doctorate and over two decades of experience in the world of hearing health. Let me be your guide through the pages of this book to circumstances of hearing loss – but more importantly, to the prospect of hearing gained through the marvelous advancements in technology.

Many people who enter my office prefer not to be here. Often they don't believe they have a problem.

If only people would speak more clearly, they say, and face them when speaking or talk loudly then they would hear much better. This book is meant to bring clarity to this sometimes misunderstood area so you can go back to enjoying the sounds of your life.

In fact, not everyone I see has a hearing problem. The most common example is wax in the ears which is easily remedied in the office. You come to an audiologist to measure your hearing, and determine if a simple fix will allow you to hear better, or diagnose the medical reason for reduced hearing.

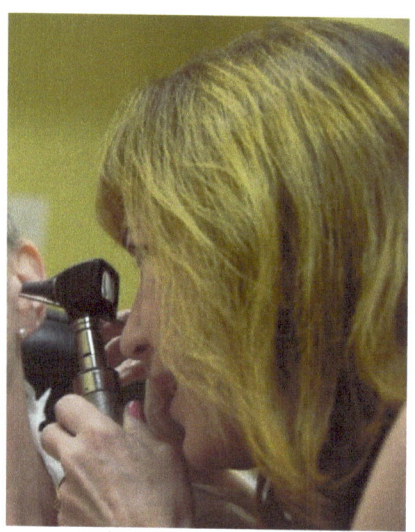

The people who come into my office usually fall into one of four categories. Only an evaluation by a professional audiologist will help you decide which category you or someone close to you belongs in.

1. **Those without a hearing deficit.** Simple errors in communication can cause the problem. Husbands and wives often relax with each other and do not speak as clearly or listen as carefully as they would with other people. They try to talk to each other from other rooms, or in areas with significant background noise. There are limits to human hearing abilities, even when ears are functioning normally.

2. **Those with earwax.** Common earwax build up can inhibit hearing, but it is fairly easily removed. Problem solved! If

this happens, they are very happy. Sometimes removing the earwax is not enough if there is also an underlying hearing problem.

3. **Those with specific treatable medical issues** that cause a loss of hearing. While involving only a small percentage of my patients, these issues can be treated with medication or surgery by an Ear, Nose and Throat physician (often called simply an ENT). I will recommend a doctor for you if your test results indicate you should see an ENT.

4. **Those with a hearing loss.** The majority of patients I evaluate have a hearing loss, significant enough to impair communications with others. With the help of an audiologist and a large range of hearing aid options, these people can significantly improve the quality of their hearing.

The fact that many patients do have a hearing loss is not surprising when you learn that hearing loss is the third most common major public health issue behind arthritis and heart disease. The Hearing Loss Association of America reports that one in five people in the United States have some degree of hearing problem. This adds up to 50 million individuals.

While hearing deficits are more common in people who are older, they can occur at any age. In fact 60 percent of those who suffer hearing loss are still in school or are working, causing a significant barrier to success in education and employment. Of every 1,000 children, two or three are hearing impaired or deaf. Untreated hearing loss causes significant failures in school and employment, decreased income over a lifetime, and may even exacerbate dementia and depression.

HOW THE AUDIOLOGIST EVALUATES HEARING

To be effective, a hearing care provider needs to get to know the patient, and to evaluate the communications environment in which the patient lives. Does the patient enjoy a very quiet lifestyle? Or is the patient a student or business person and highly dependent on every word that is said? Is the patient highly extroverted e.g. someone that frequents noisy restaurants, parties or sporting events? This information is especially meaningful for diagnosis and treatment. A history of noise exposure is particularly relevant. People who have been exposed to significant or prolonged noise exposure such as gun use, construction equipment, or in the service are much more likely to have a permanent hearing loss.

As with other medical professionals you may visit, past medical history unrelated to the ears is also key for making an informed diagnosis. We will use an otoscope to look into your ears to evaluate the ear canal and eardrum.

After we understand your medical history and inspect your ears, we will test your hearing which is perhaps the most crucial aspect of the visit.

In an audiologist's office you'll find a sound proof room where the hearing test is performed. Sitting in the sound proof room wearing headphones, you will listen to tones through the headphones, and push a button every time you hear a tone. The tone levels are varied to discover the limits of your hearing capabilities.

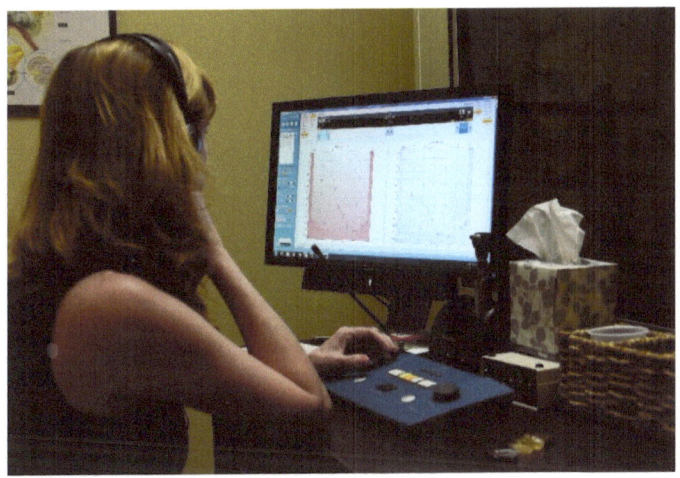

This test of tones is repeated several times at different frequencies to allow us to determine the very softest level that the patient can barely hear. This level of sound is called a threshold. Think of a threshold of a doorway; it is the difference between being in the room and being outside of the room. For hearing, the difference is between hearing nothing and hearing something no matter how small. Many people worry about how they are doing on this test, due to the fact that the sound is so soft they are unsure if they heard it – but the test is in fact designed to find this level.

Next, the patient's ability to hear and understand speech is evaluated. This speech test is intended to validate the findings of the threshold tone test. The patient repeats words that gradually are spoken more softly, until they are no longer heard.

A secondary speech test seeks to determine the level in which you comfortably hear speech and how well you can understand words. We achieve this based on the results of the previous tonal exam and adjusting the speech level you hear through headphones. If you score high on this test, speech sounds are clear to you, and you will be more successful with hearing aids as compared to someone who has a difficult time understanding speech, even if it is at a sufficient volume. This test also gives the audiologist more information on the health of the inner ear.

Next comes a test of bone conduction. Why? Hearing depends on how well the inner ear -- the mechanism for hearing -- works. To determine the workings of the inner ear a headband is positioned against the skull (the mastoid bone) to deliver different frequency vibrations that can be compared to the thresholds through headphones. If sound is heard much better through the bone conductor, then it is possible that medical treatment could improve hearing. The testing results for the patient are called an audiogram. The audiogram is an evaluation of the patient's hearing abilities, although it does not really tell us how the hearing loss affects the individual's life skills.

If there is a hearing problem, what are the probable causes? Is there a possible medical treatment that can improve the patient's hearing? If there is, I refer you to an ENT for further evaluation and treatment. Audiologists have a close working relationship with ENTs. The ENT needs our hearing evaluations to evaluate you medically.

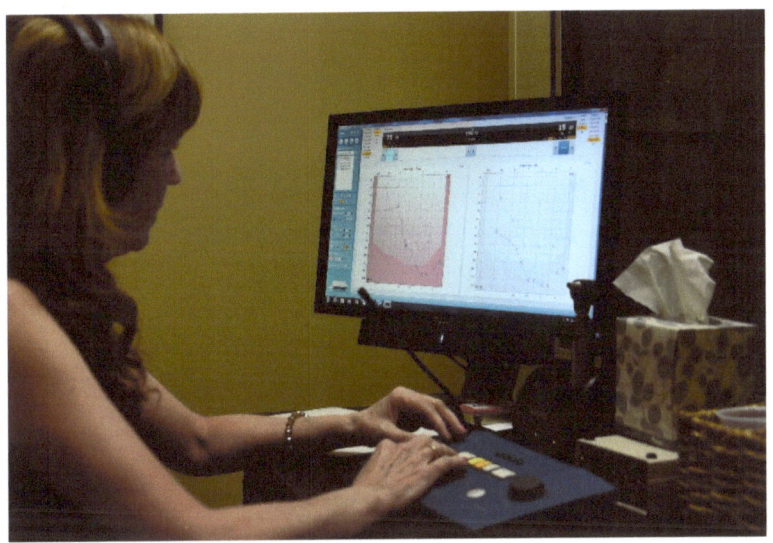

DEVICES AND TREATMENTS FOR HEARING LOSS

Common treatments once hearing loss is diagnosed:

- The use of hearing aids or other devices that amplify sound

- Devices such as cochlear implants that convert sound to an electrical impulse to stimulate the inner ear when hearing aids are not enough to improve communication

- Modifications in communication environments such as moving a person closer to those who are speaking (preferential seating in the classroom or a meeting, getting people to face you while they are speaking)

- Room amplifiers with microphones and speakers (these may be used for a child with a mild hearing loss in a classroom)

- Captions or subtitles

- Headphones such as TV Ears, to view television

- Medical treatments such as medication or surgery
- Vitamin supplements and other holistic treatments have been recommended by some to diminish or reverse the effects of hearing loss

Most people who have a hearing loss don't need an ENT—they will benefit from hearing aids.

2 – HEARING LOSS AND BEHAVIORAL EFFECTS

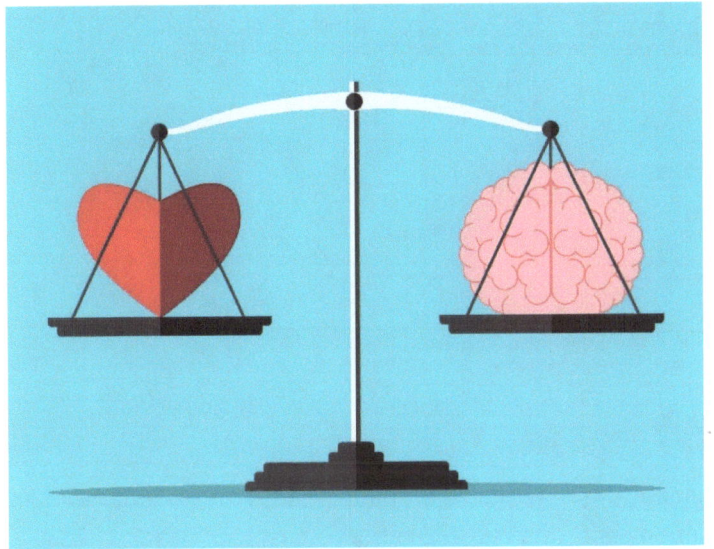

The initial stages of a hearing loss can be discouraging and confusing. Are people mumbling? My spouse could turn around when she is speaking? Or is she turning away from me deliberately? **Am I getting old?** Are people talking faster than they used to? **Am I turning into my grandfather**? It can be quite embarrassing when the person with the hearing loss misunderstands what is said to them.

For a person who is not aware of the circumstances brought on by a hearing loss, the emotional effects may be devastating!

Is the hearing problem a result of aging? Did I spend too much time listening to loud music or shooting guns? Did I fail to protect my hearing? Or is there a physical cause that may be medically evaluated or treated? (For further discussion on medical causes or hearing loss, see Chapter 4.)

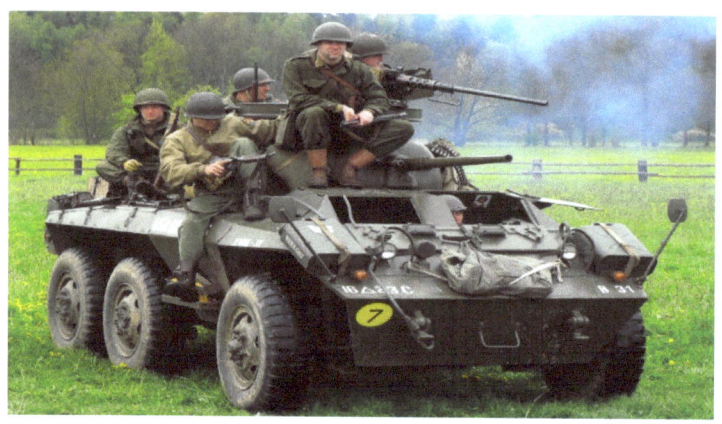

Thank you for your service, unfortunately guns and hearing are not a good mix

Fortunately, for veterans, the United States government has developed programs that will help veterans with hearing loss or tinnitus (ringing in the ears) that causes a significant disability. If you are a veteran and unable to obtain services for your hearing, talk to your local Veteran's administration who will give you more information on the programs that are available including payment for hearing aids and services, and monthly payments for service connected disabilities. In the more recent past, the VA has contracted with local audiology offices to handle the deluge of veterans needing assistance with their hearing. Ask your local audiologist for information.

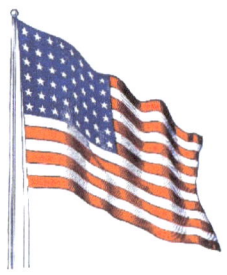

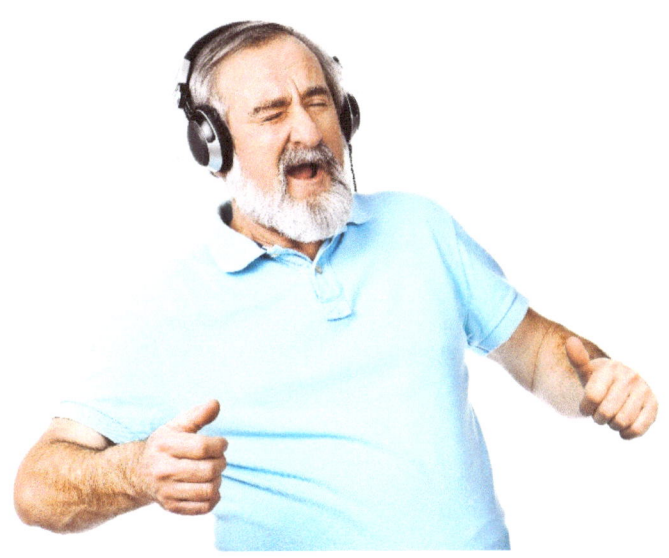

Loud Music - all fun and games until someone damages their hearing!

Hearing loss is associated with an increased incidence of depression, isolation, and dementia. Dr. Frank Lin from Johns Hopkins in Baltimore has been studying the side effects of hearing loss for years as part of the Baltimore Longitudinal Study of Aging. In addition to depression and dementia, some people experience paranoia since they don't realize that the problem is theirs and not that others are making communication more difficult for them. Because hearing difficulties make social situations challenging and frustrating, many people avoid them which further separates them from other people. These are major, debilitating factors.

Co-dependent behavior of someone suffering hearing loss is a frequent and often difficult situation prolonging necessary treatment. When the spouse helps translate a conversation, the spouse with the hearing loss may be able to get by more easily and this encourages denial. The hearing spouse helps order in a restaurant, or makes sure the person who cannot hear clearly understands what is going on in a group situation. The hearing spouse is trying to help the loved one, but slows down the realization by the spouse who needs treatment.

A hearing loss is not just a physical problem; it has an effect on **all relationships and interactions**. The feelings related to hearing loss are important to explore by talking to your audiologist or hearing care provider, a sympathetic friend, family member, clergy or a professional in the psychology field.

As an audiologist, it may come as no surprise that I also recommend properly fit hearing aids. When fit well by a professional hearing care provider, the devices go far to diminish the emotional concerns associated with hearing problems.

- Hearing aids are always less obvious than "What?" or "Huh?"
- Understanding a conversation makes you appear more intelligent
- People who hear well have happier relationships
- Social activities are more enjoyable if you can hear better
- Less worry of embarrassment from misunderstanding conversation
- Reduced anxiety related to hearing and safety

How can hearing devices help us and just how do they work? Let's explore this in the following chapters.

3 – SO I NEED A HEARING AID, NOW WHAT?

If the hearing evaluation determines the need for hearing aids, we use the following three criteria to hone in on the right type of hearing device: **style, performance, and cost.**

Style

Style refers to the type of hearing aid.

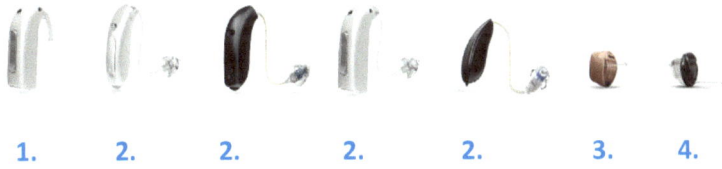

1.   2.   2.   2.   2.   3.   4.

1. Behind the ear - BTE
2. Receiver in the ear - RITE (various styles or sizes)
3. Completely in the canal - CIC
4. Invisible in canal - IIC

- **Behind-the-ear (BTE)** – As the name implies, the entire device is located over the ear. Then a custom made earmold is attached which sends the sound into the ear. This device provides the most power for people who need it, and is suitable for people with middle ear problems resulting in perforations or drainage. This hearing aid is more visible than the RITE. Directional microphones help to provide better hearing in noisy environments.

- **Receiver in the ear** – Currently the most popular style. This type of device has a fairly small hearing aid over the ear that hides fairly well behind the ear, and a thin wire that runs down into the ear. This is a fairly well concealed hearing aid, especially for anyone with some hair. It often provides for more comfortable hearing of the person's voice, and better hearing in noise due to the use of directional microphones.

- **Completely-in-the-canal and invisible-in-canal** -When the hearing aid user is interested in keeping the hearing device very small and the least visible, these styles are sometimes chosen. They do not contain directional microphones the BTE and RITE do because of their small size. Sometimes these devices can cause the hearing aid wearer's own voice to sound strange, which can bother some users depending on their hearing levels. These small styles are very small which means changing batteries more frequently and cleaning may be more difficult for some. On the other hand, holding a phone to your ear, or using a stethoscope may be easier with this style. Ask your audiologist for advice on these issues. Fairly recently, these devices have been equipped with features that allow the user to adjust them and use them with Bluetooth devices.

- **In-the-ear and canal hearing aids** - are custom made to the ear. They are not used as often anymore, but some people still want them. These devices have directional microphones to help hearing in noise.

- **Bone-anchored-hearing-aid (BAHA)** - were designed to help people who have severe problems with the middle ear. These could be ossicles (middle ear bones) that may not be able to be repaired, tumors or large cysts in that area, or birth defects causing a child to have no ear canal. A BAHA device is also used at times when the person has no hearing in one ear. The BAHA vibrates when sound is presented to the microphones; this vibration causes the skull to vibrate sending the sound directly to the cochlea (inner ear) and provides much improved hearing for those with this type of problem. Some users of BAHA hearing devices wear this device on a small implanted post behind the ear, others on a small magnet implanted under the skin behind the ear. Others, especially small children, wear the device on a headband holding it close enough the mastoid bone to send sounds to the cochlea.

- **Cochlear Implants -** When hearing aids can no longer help the person hear better, due to the severity of the hearing loss, a cochlear implant may be used to help the patient with communication. The cochlear implant is a special device that allows the patient to "hear" with electronic impulses delivered to the cochlea (inner ear). The cochlear implant in the diagram, involves surgery

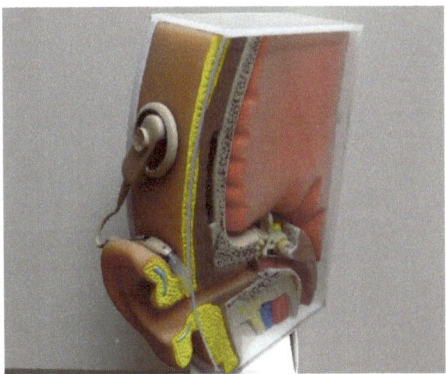 where an electrode is threaded into the cochlea. The sound processor is then programmed by an audiologist specially trained for this type of device. This audiologist may be found at the facility doing the surgery, or at a few local clinics.

Performance

Performance means the level of control in hearing aids. In other words, the ability to alter the program set-up to accommodate different noise environments, buttons to increase or decrease volume, connectivity so as to listen to devices like your television or telephone, and even the internet directly into your ears. Performance also refers to noise reduction and other types of adjustment that operate without you knowing to help you hear the best possible.

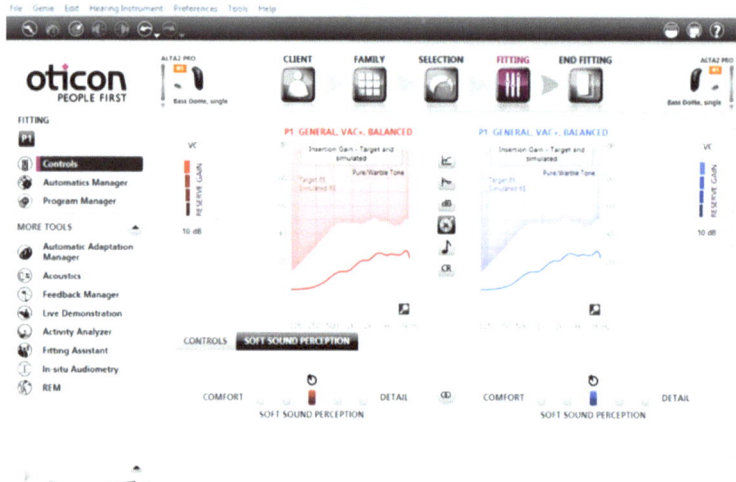

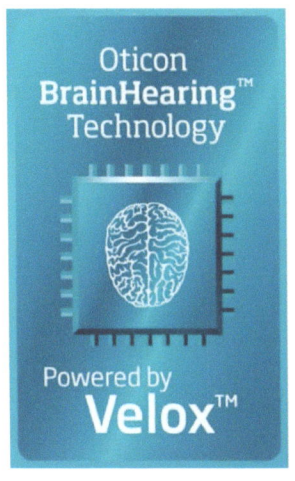

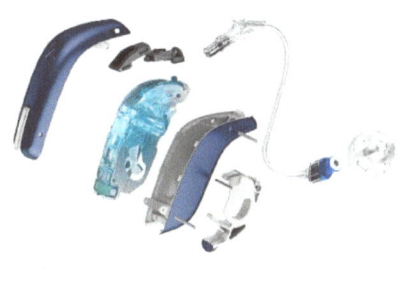

Hearing aids contain microprocessors that work to boost the desired sounds like speech and filter out the background noise.

Most hearing aids are capable of Bluetooth connections now. In premium hearing devices, there are also features such as automatic speech guard and the latest in background noise reduction. The premium hearing devices contain all the bells and whistles. Some people think they do not need the additional technical advantages – but they can free you from needing to make frequent

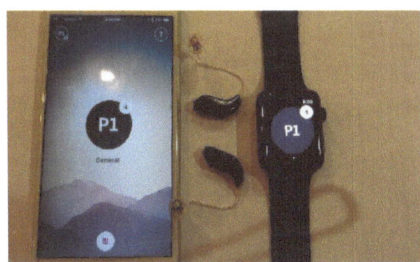

Bells and whistles, include hearing aids that can be connected to your iPhone and controlled by the phone or even your Apple watch!

manual changes in volume or programs to the hearing aid since they are already being made automatically - thus making the devices simpler to use.

Maybe you don't want all the bells -- and with hearing aids you certainly don't want whistles! Okay, that's an audiology joke—hearing aids sometimes whistle and we have to correct for that-- but you get the picture. With the guidance of your audiologist you must decide what you want your hearing aids to do.

Newer hearing devices can be programmed to reduce background noise and enhance speech as well as be customized for the individual patient's needs in a variety of situations.

Cost

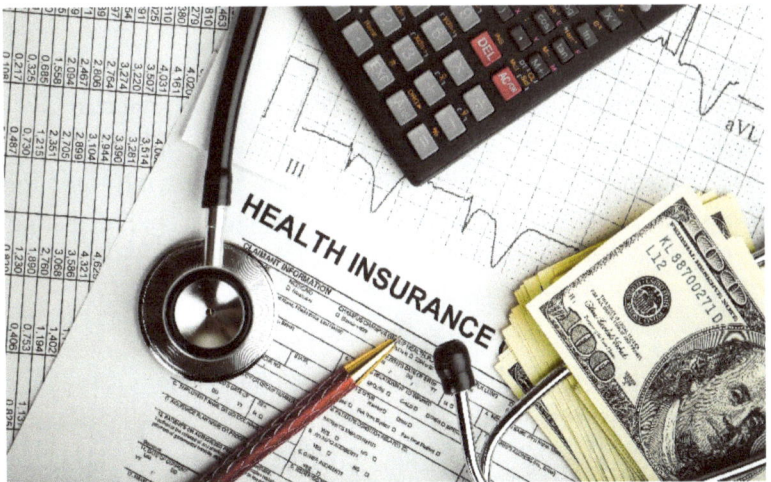

Our goal is to provide the best hearing aid for your budget which may not be the newest technology or most expensive hearing aid. While we make every effort to have hearing aids covered by medical insurance the reality is that they are not commonly covered. For those that are covered by insurance for hearing devices, the employer is usually the reason. A few that we have found that have some coverage for hearing aids in our area include Los Angeles Unified School District, Motion Picture and Screen Actors' Guild, Federal or State Employees, and Los Angeles Police Department employees and families. Ask your audiologist or insurance company for more information on potential coverage.

Many audiologists include their on-going services with the cost of the hearing aids so that the patient has the ability to have the hearing aids cleaned or adjusted as needed with no additional cost for a period of years. Others "unbundle" the charges allowing the hearing aid user to pay a lower cost for the hearing aids, then pay for follow up visits as they go.

New users of hearing devices may not realize how important this level of service is. They think that they are buying a radio to take home and use. Once a person starts using hearing aids, they find how valuable it is in improving his or her life and want to keep the aids in tip-top shape. In a full service audiology office, the hearing aid user can be assured the devices will be maintained properly.

This is not to suggest that each person will have regular issues with his or her hearing aids, however, maintenance and problem situations do arise. The user may go to the audiologist with a problem and get a simple repair in a few minutes. Hearing aid cleaning is very important and neglected at times, so hearing aid filters and microphones may become plugged and need maintenance. If the problem is larger, the hearing aid may be sent for repair and the patient fit with a loaner so there is no interruption in hearing. The audiologist also calls the patient back into the office for testing and adjustments to accommodate small changes in hearing before they become a problem.

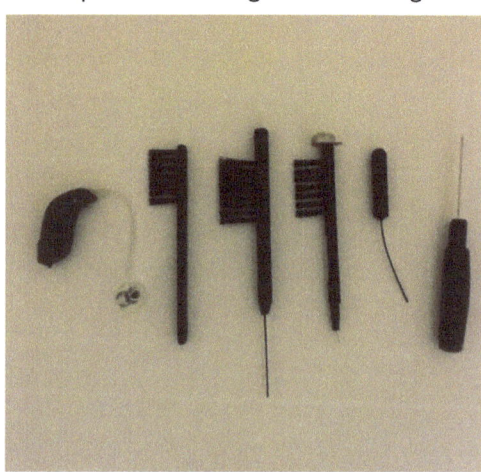

A few examples of the cleaning tools available with the hearing device

This degree of service adds to the cost of hearing aids. The benefit of this system is that the person wearing

25

hearing aids is more likely to be happy with the hearing aids they are using if they can visit the audiologist whenever they feel the need without additional costs for each visit. Many individuals would be less likely to make additional required visits for needed adjustments and assistance if they know each visit will be charged, so an **'all inclusive'** plan which includes all the follow up care required provides the best alternative for many patients. Even though this is what the audiologist recommends, discuss your concerns about cost with the provider, they may be able to make different arrangements to help you hear better right away.

It is important to keep in mind that a hearing aid is a medical device that should be fit by a medical professional and therefore cannot be compared to the costs associated with going to a store to purchase consumer devices such as smart phones or home entertainment systems.

Modern hearing devices are programmed to a patient's needs with complex computerized fitting programs allowing for manipulation of literally thousands of customized parameters. The combination of technology and the well-trained hearing provider's experience truly make hearing health care and the job of an audiologist a blend of art and science.

CONSUMER BEWARE!

Be aware that there are devices called **personal amplifiers** available on the market that cause some confusion with people needing hearing aids. These devices are generally available by mail order, partly due to the fact that laws govern the sale of fitting devices to protect consumers.

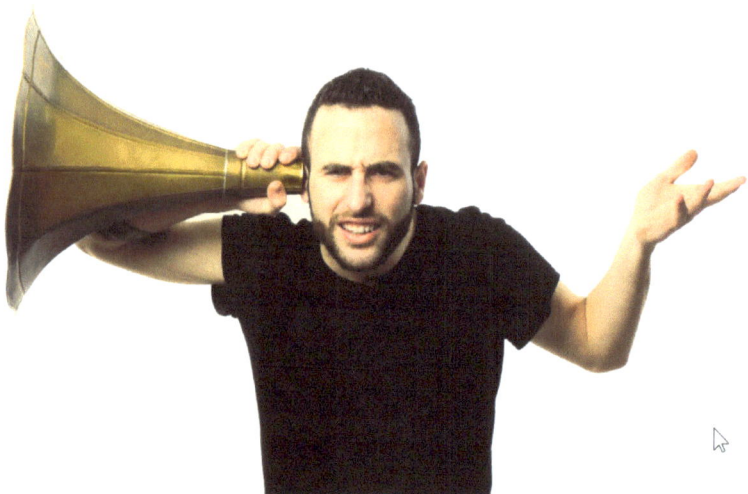

By ordering such devices without visiting an audiologist, users typically do not have a hearing test. They do not know if they simply have wax in their ears or something more serious like a perforated eardrum causes the hearing problem. Results of the hearing test that would indicate the type of hearing loss that would benefit from medical treatment are not identified, so this treatment does not occur.

The devices are sent in the mail with limited instructions so the user has to learn how to insert the devices, change the battery, and learn how to clean the aids by themselves. They are also sold at some pharmacy stores as if they were reading glasses.

Settings on the devices are set at an estimated level without a hearing test – this is like buying glasses for a more complicated vision problem without a vision test. Hearing aid levels should be set corresponding to the hearing loss pitch.

Unfortunately, many people using this type of device are not helped to hear well, so they develop a negative attitude about hearing aids. They are upset because they wasted money and still have a problem.

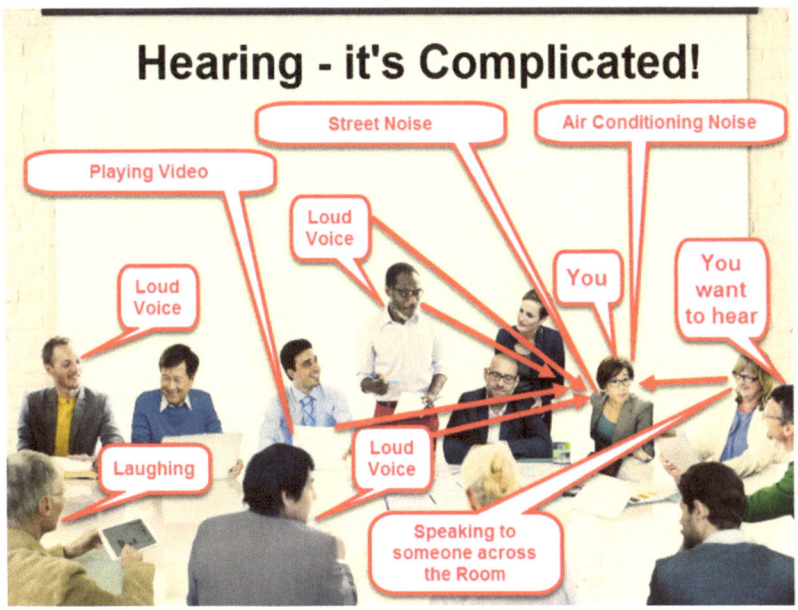

4 – THE BASICS OF HEARING LOSS AND HEARING DEVICES

A BRIEF HISTORY OF HEARING DEVICES

Imagine what Beethoven, the famously deaf composer, or Helen Keller, the well-known deaf-blind humanitarian who was the first with her conditions to earn a bachelor's degree, could have done with modern day hearing aids. From ear trumpets to electronic hearing aids that were so large they would be carried in a wagon, sound amplification has been through an evolutionary process that has soared to new heights lately.

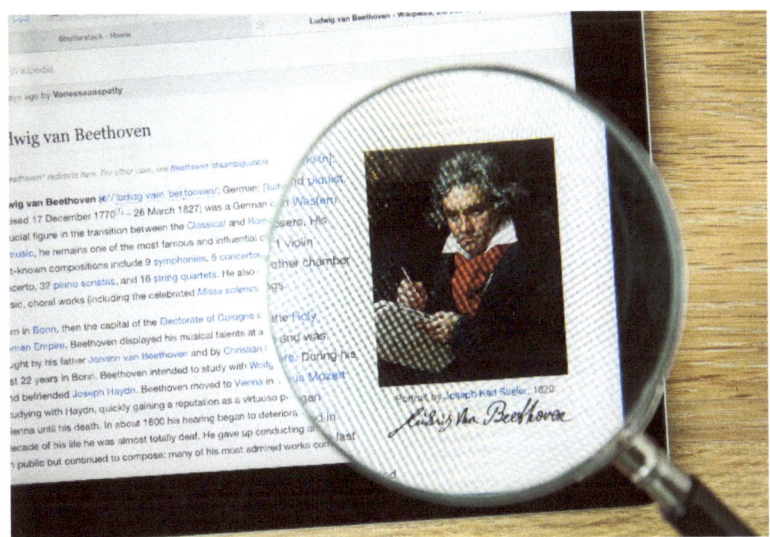

The first and a very simple way of increasing a sound to the ear was a cupped hand against the ear increasing the loudness of speech. Ear trumpets were popular for many years during the

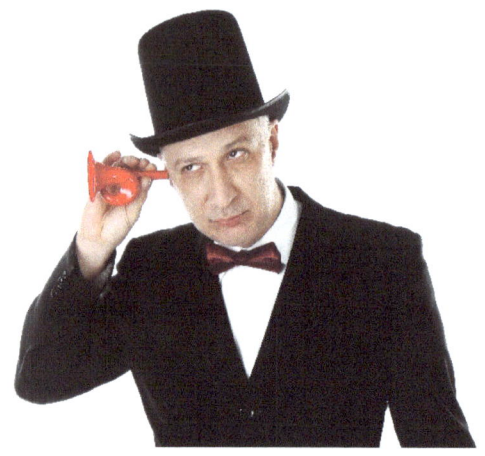

1800s to early 1900s. Body hearing aids were fairly large devices, worn around the wearer's neck or chest. They were used for more severe hearing losses throughout the 20th century. Later, hearing aids were developed to be worn behind the ear or in the ear. Some hearing aids were even incorporated with eyeglass frames

All hearing devices, whether they are analog or digital and regardless of the manufacturer that produces them consist of a few specific components: the microphone, the amplifier, and the receiver. More on how hearing aids work in chapter 5.

Analog hearing aids are generally obsolete, but still occasionally used. The devices use simple amplification of sound waves so they boost all sounds (speech and noise). Unfortunately, background sounds are amplified as well, which inhibits understanding of speech.

The big breakthrough for hearing aid technology came in 1996 when hearing devices became fully computer programmable and digital. **Digital hearing aids** are able to do a much better job treating hearing loss. All sounds picked up by the microphones of these hearing aids are converted to digital signals. After they are converted, the sounds may be manipulated in a much greater way than analog hearing aids were able to.

Today, hearing devices can be mostly concealed by hair near the ears. The devices are manufactured in varying colors to blend in.

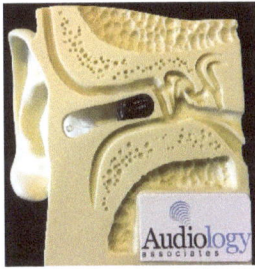

Other people choose to have devices that are completely invisible – they are worn deep in the ear canal. Some choose to have fun when selecting hearing aids, choosing attractive colors (more children than adults). **Honestly, the best device is the one that the patient is comfortable wearing, and is able to use to hear well.**

IIC Hearing Device

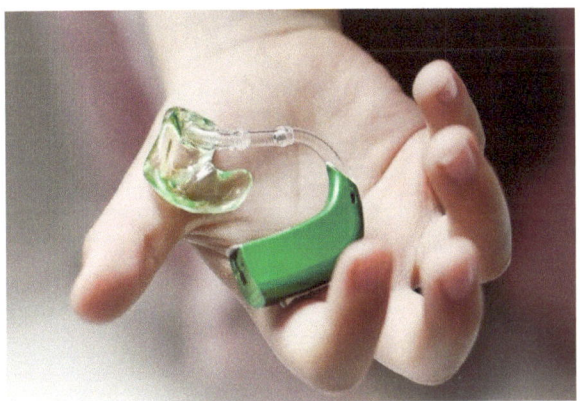

While the device color can blend in with the hair and scalp some choose a 'fun' and colorful device

A SIMPLIFIED DISCUSSION OF THE EAR ANATOMY

The human ear is an amazing system – extremely small and encased in the bones of the skull. It is a complex structure. Let's take a quick journey through the human ear.

- The **outer ear** contains the visible part of the ear made up of cartilage and skin and is designed to capture sound.
- Follow along through the cave-like **ear canal** that leads to the **eardrum** (tympanic membrane). Our journey may be made difficult because we have to work our way through ear wax (cerumen) that can build up and block sound from entering the ear.

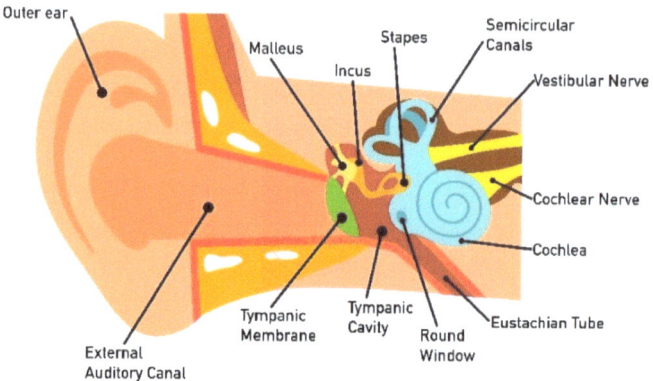

- Next comes the **middle ear**. The eardrum is attached to three small bones in a chain with joints, similar to the bones in your finger. They are the three smallest bones in the body. Their job is to act like pistons to transfer and amplify the sound to the inner ear.
- Connected to the middle ear is the **Eustachian tube**. The purpose of this tube is to equalize the pressure in the middle ear with changes of altitude for comfort and hearing. If this tube malfunctions, hearing changes occur and pain or pressure in the ear follow. You may have experienced some of that pain as an airplane descends for a landing. Young children and babies usually do. That's why you'll often hear them crying as a plane lands.
- Sound now reaches the **inner ear**. The inner ear, or the **cochlea**, is often described as looking like a snail shell

33

(cochlea is Greek for spiral or snail shell). It is the most complex part of the hearing system and is the organ of hearing. It contains thousands of nerve cells (very small nerves, called inner and outer hair cells). These hair cells cause the nerve to identify a sound and send that sound on its way ending in the auditory cortex of the brain.

Think of the inner ear as the gatekeeper to the brain

This amazing process gives specific information to the brain with the type of sound or combination of sounds that is heard. When the system is working well, extremely complex combinations of sounds are discerned, for example understanding speech from a few different people at the same time even over background noise. The astute listener can hear musical sounds including many instruments playing in an orchestra, and possibly even hear which instruments are out of tune.

ONE IMPORTANT WARNING!

Noise induced hearing loss is a major cause of hearing loss that is entirely preventable. Wear ear protection when

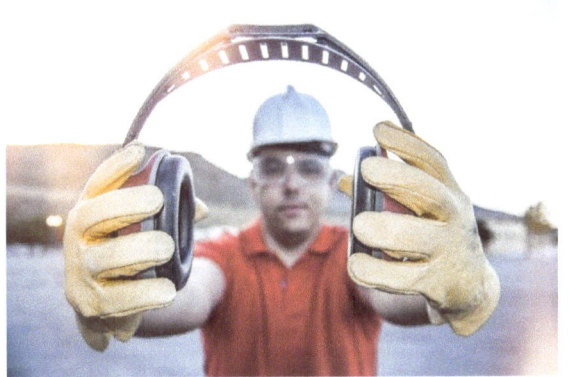

necessary, and reduce your time being exposed to these loud sounds as much as possible. If you are using power tools, shooting firearms, mowing the lawn or involved in other very noisy environments – the key to when you need ear protection is if you need to raise your voice to be heard. Veterans, police officers, firefighters, and many who work in industrial environments develop permanent hearing loss, and were sometimes in the difficult situation of being unable to do their jobs at the same time as properly protecting their ears.

The **inner** and **outer hair cells** do not regenerate. Unfortunately, this means that once a hair cell is damaged by noise exposure, age, genetic changes to the ear, or disease these nerves will never regrow. The cells are set up like a piano as far as tones, so in the photograph below, a large part of the "keyboard" is

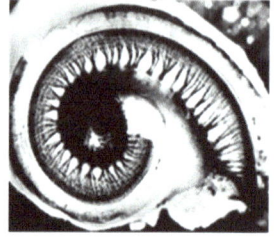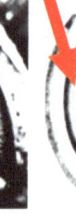

missing. These are sounds the person will never hear.

Normal Cochlear   Damaged Cochlear

DISEASES AND THE IMPORTANCE OF EARLY TESTING

There are many diseases that are associated with hearing loss. Some such as shingles or meningitis (which may cause deafness) may be avoided with vaccinations. Others need to be recognized as part of several medical symptoms that need treatment.

Meniere's disease causes frequent vertigo and fluctuations in hearing, usually only on one side. The person who has this is often very sick and affected by the hearing loss, but also by vertigo, intermittent ringing in the ears, and fluctuating hearing. An audiologist will evaluate hearing, but the person is usually treated by a neurologist or ENT. Hearing aids may be used to treat the hearing loss.

Genetic disorders are a common cause of hearing loss. Some patients will tell me that most or all of the people in their family are hard of hearing. Just like other genetic traits such as blue eyes, or long legs, hearing loss may be in your genes. There are numerous hereditary conditions causing hearing problems, some related to other systems in the body such as eyes, skin or kidneys and others that involve only the ears. About half of all hearing loss is genetic although a portion of that is *presbycusis*-- the loss of hearing that gradually occurs in many individuals as they grow older. In other words, while some families have gray hair at earlier ages, others have hearing loss before reaching older age.

I know a veteran who suffers with Usher's syndrome which causes a progressive hearing loss and a loss of vision. He enlisted in the army in spite of a hearing problem, and discovered the vision problem later on. He has been an inspiration since he provides counseling to veterans with different types of disabilities that have occurred while they served their country. Dealing with a hearing loss in a positive way is very important to balance negative feelings.

Much as muscles benefit from exercise, the split second processing the human brain undertakes to evaluate and understand speech takes practice and training. Think of hearing aids as a workout aid for the imaginary ear muscle. If the brain stops receiving stimulation, it gets 'out of shape' causing the mind to became weak.

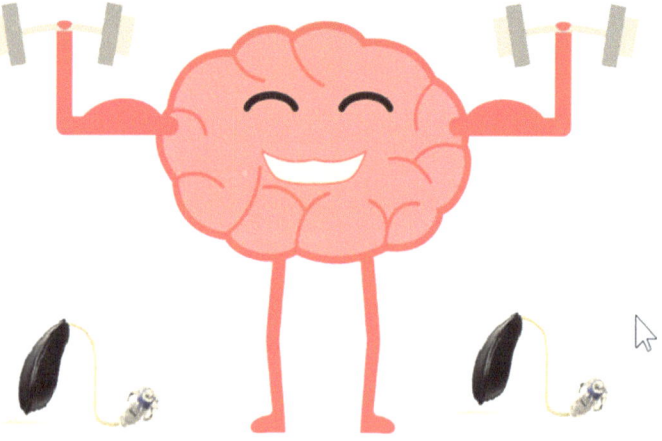

Your Brain needs to keep exercising to stay in top shape!
Your ears help provide the workout.

If you are not hearing well, your brain won't get enough exercise!

Brain Health - On a more academic note, Frank Lin, MD, PhD, an otologist and epidemiologist at Johns Hopkins in Baltimore reports his findings of major studies that show that hearing plays a much more important role in brain health than medicine has traditionally believed.

Dr. Lin reported that older adults with mild hearing loss have twice the incidence of dementia as compared with those without hearing loss. Moderate to severe hearing loss is accompanied by three to four times the incidence of dementia.

Although the reasons for the increase in dementia are not definite, Doctors Lin, Metter, O'Brien and others report that causes for the increased levels of dementia fall into four general categories:

1. Associated medical problems that may affect hearing and cognition (such as high blood pressure).
2. Increased cognitive load caused by working harder to understand what people are saying.
3. Hearing loss may affect brain structure in a way that contributes to cognitive problems.
4. Social isolation. Being socially isolated has long been recognized as a risk factor for cognitive decline.

That information is disturbing, but encouragingly, hearing impaired people who use hearing aids regularly have dementia at basically the same rate as those with normal hearing.   Why is this the case? Realize that people with hearing loss have to work harder at communication than those with normal hearing. Because these situations are more difficult, many people avoid complex work and social activities. Hearing impaired individuals who use hearing aids are much more able to participate in life and they benefit from this participation.

Untreated hearing loss also increases the likelihood of depression, isolation, paranoia, insecurity, and can cause negative effects on a variety of medical health conditions, too.

Because of the damage that untreated hearing loss can do, and the problem with gradual hearing loss being unnoticed or denied, it would be wise to catch the condition earlier rather than later. Screening for hearing loss should begin in young adulthood (a baseline by age 40), particularly for vulnerable groups, such as diabetics.

Please review this important study regarding the relationship between hearing loss and cognitive decline:

New Study Shows Hearing Aids Reduce Risk of Cognitive Decline in Older Adults

hearingreview.com/2015/10/new-study-shows-hearing-aids-reduce-risk-of-cognitive-decline-in-older-adults/

A new long-term study that shows wearing hearing aids to reduce cognitive decline associated with hearing loss may do more than just drive older adults with hearing loss to finally seek professional care, according to Oticon. The company believes the new study will also give the general public—especially health-conscious older adults—a new way of thinking about the importance of hearing care and hearing solutions that will have far-reaching implications for hearing care now and in the future.

"Self-Reported Hearing Loss: Hearing Aids and Cognitive Decline in Elderly Adults: A 25-year Study," published in the October edition of the Journal of the American Geriatrics Society compared the trajectory of cognitive decline among older adults who were using hearing aids and those who were not. The study found no difference in the rate of cognitive decline between a control group of people with no reported hearing loss and people with hearing loss who used hearing aids. By contrast, untreated hearing loss was significantly associated with lower baseline scores on the Mini-Mental State Examination, a well-established test of cognitive function, during the 25-year follow-up period, independent of age, gender, and education.

Hélène Amieva, PhD
Professor *Hélène Amieva*, a leading researcher in the Neuropsychology and Epidemiology of Aging at the University of Bordeaux, France, headed up the study which followed 3,670 adults age 65 and older over a 25-year period as part of the Personnes Agèes QUID cohort (PAQUID), a cohort specifically designed to study brain aging. Professor Amieva shared the study's early findings at *Oticon's 2014 OtiCongress*, a knowledge-sharing event that explored cognitive health and the benefits of Oticon's *BrainHearing™* technology.

Donald Schum, PhD
"Improved communication made possible by hearing aids resulted in improved mood, social interactions and cognitively stimulating abilities and is the most likely underlying reason for the decreased cognitive decline reported in the study," says Donald Schum, PhD, vice president of Audiology and Professional Relations for Oticon Inc. *"For nearly 20 years, Oticon researchers at the Eriksholm research center have focused on the development of BrainHearing technologies that help the brain make sense of sound so that people with a hearing impairment can maintain or regain the ability and mental*

The study findings strengthen our energy to engage socially. commitment to a "brain first" approach to designing hearing solutions."

Helping the Brain Make Sense of Sound
Rather than emphasize amplification and suppression of sounds, Oticon reports that its "brain first" audiological approach recognizes that speech understanding and comprehension are cognitive processes that happen in the brain. According to the company, the Inium Sense platform supports BrainHearing technology so that wearers can enjoy a fit personalized to their unique hearing loss and sound preferences for a more natural listening experience and better speech understanding with less effort.

"By targeting research on performance, effort, and energy demand, we continue to develop new hearing solutions that enable wearers to preserve energy throughout the day so they can engage more actively in everyday life," explains Schum.

Hearing solutions with BrainHearing technologies deliver a 96% satisfaction rating for both experienced and first time wearers when compared with a 79% industry average for typical hearing aids currently being fit to patients, according to Oticon.

Hearing Care is Health Care
The potential for the findings of the PAQUID study to increase focus on hearing health care within the broader context of health care for healthy aging is considerable.

Beyond the immediate reach to the American Geriatric Society's 6,000 geriatrics and gerontological health professionals, the study findings will influence other health care professionals charged with improving the health, independence and quality of life of people as they age.

Oticon encourages hearing care professionals to explain the health risk of untreated hearing loss to patients as a way of motivating them to do the right thing to treat their hearing loss. "Cognitive health is a concern across all age groups but especially among older adults," says Schum. "The PAQUID study is very important news for those people who are considering doing something about treating their hearing loss but have been delaying. It's not just about hearing well today, it's about the long-term effects of untreated hearing loss."

Oticon has developed educational and community outreach materials to support hearing care professionals in increasing awareness of the connection between hearing, hearing solutions and cognition among patients and other health care practitioners in their communities.

For more information on hearing loss, cognition, and BrainHearing technology, visit brainhearing.com.

Additionally, in the September 2015 edition of The Hearing Review, Oticon Director of Professional Relations Douglas Beck, PhD, guest-edited a series of articles titled "Expert Roundtable: Cognition, Audition, and Amplification: 2015" that includes perspectives from leading experts in hearing care research.
Source: Oticon

hearingreview.com/2015/10/new-study-shows-hearing-aids-reduce-risk-of-cognitive-decline-in-older-adults/

5 – HOW HEARING AIDS WORK

They are Magic!

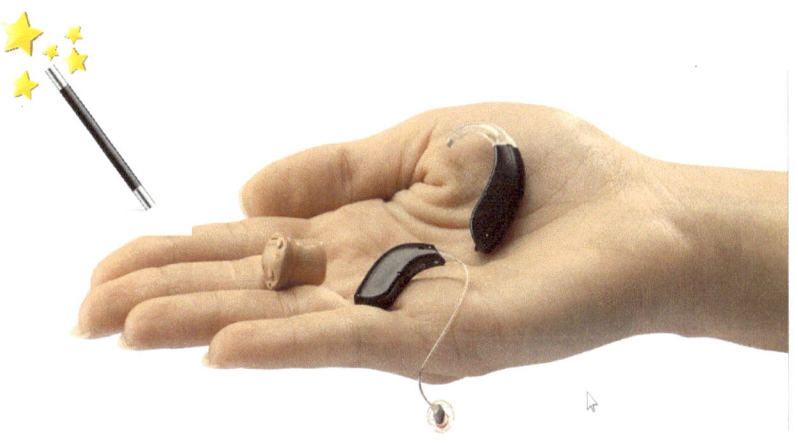

Hearing aids are devices that help improve sound perception. When a person has a hearing loss, they lose the ability to hear some frequencies or pitches of the sound range. For most people with difficulty hearing, consonant sounds are more difficult to discern. Sounds such *as s, t, sh, ch, f, h, th, p*, etc. are hard or impossible to hear, unless they are amplified.

Some words that would easily be misunderstood are:

- sixty, fifty – fifteenth, fiftieth
- sixteen, fifteen
- eight, ace, eighth, ache
- car, scar, tar, far
- six, fix, chicks
- tap, chap, chat, cat, slap
- talk, chalk, stop
- cheap, sheep, seep

For instance, a person may hear "fifty dollars and sixty-six cents" and start writing a check, instead of the correct: "sixty dollars and fifty-six cents." Ninety percent of the power of speech is in the low frequencies, yet ninety percent of the understanding of speech in the high frequencies. The higher frequencies are almost always the part of hearing that is lost first.

Hearing loss differs from vision loss

As with the eye, the ear's performance is affected by aging. However, bad vision gradually makes reading harder as the letters get smaller, but hearing loss is different.

Hearing loss can make certain syllables and sounds harder to hear. For example, high-pitched consonants like f, s and t are easily drowned out by louder, low-pitched vowels like a, o and u. This results in a person with hearing loss complaining that they can hear others are talking, but not what they are saying.

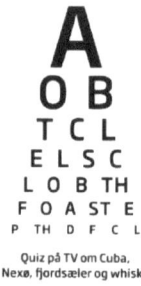

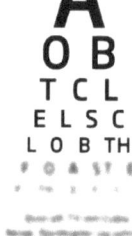

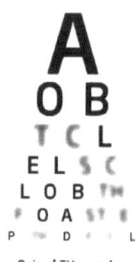

| Normal hearing | Visual impairment | Hearing impairment |

Missing sounds that are parts of words change or remove all meaning from conversations and leaves the listener lost and out of the conversation

As was previously mentioned, this causes the person with hearing loss to be continually trying to figure out what is said by the context of the sentence, or trying to lip-read the missing letters. The listener may also fall behind in the conversation taking that extra time to decipher what was said. Once the listener is behind, it is nearly impossible to catch up since there is a continuous flow of new words that may also be missed.

Hearing aids can be adjusted to make up for most of the power deficiencies and understanding speech. Hearing aids are designed with a potential range of power levels by the manufacturer of the device. The major manufacturers in the United States are: **Oticon, Starkey, Phonak, Widex, Resound and Siemens, Rexton, and Bernafon**. Within the range of power levels, there are many other features available with regard to size, placement, appearance, and other features related to sound quality. As hearing aids evolve and advances in new features are released, some manufacturers will provide hearing aids that are more commonly used. Your hearing care provider can give you more guidance in this decision.

A device is chosen by the audiologist and patient based on the hearing levels and the specific listening needs and financial expectations of the patient. Several factors are considered such as the degree of hearing loss, background noise reduction needs, Bluetooth connectivity, size and appearance of the device and many other advanced features that may help to distinguish the desired speech signal from the unwanted background noise. Then the hearing instrument is customized further by the hearing practitioner based on the results of the audiogram, and many other requested features. The provider will probably let you try more than one to compare if you choose.

Hearing devices consist of a few main components: the **microphone**, the **amplifier**, and the **receiver**. These devices may be digital or analog. Most are digital now.

Microphone: All sounds are picked up by the microphone of a hearing aid and directed to the **amplifier** which "amplifies" the sound so that the user may hear it. The amount of amplification depends on what the audiologist and manufacturer have selected for the specific hearing aid and listener. The **receiver,** sometimes referred to as the **speaker,** delivers the amplified sound to the patient's ear. There are a variety of ways this may occur such as through an earmold, an in the ear speaker or hearing aid.

Analog hearing aids are generally obsolete, but deserve a basic description. The process involves simple amplification of sound waves so they boost all sounds (speech and noise). This allows the listener to hear sounds that were not loud enough to hear. Amplification could be provided to speech, but did not include as many high frequency sounds. Analog hearing aids used a system called "peak clipping" which reduces loud sounds, but provide a degree of distortion to sounds. Unfortunately, background sounds are amplified as well, which inhibits understanding of speech.

Digital hearing instruments are the other main type. Aside from a few models, almost all hearing aids presently fit are digital, since the huge technology transition in 1996. For digital hearing aids, a computer chip inside the hearing aid is coded with the requirements of the hearing aid user based on their specific hearing needs and the modifications that the audiologist and the hearing aid user make together. Digital hearing aids are capable of processing higher frequency speech sounds

All sounds picked up by the microphones of these hearing aids are converted by a tiny device in the hearing aid called an **analog to digital converter**. After they are converted, the sounds may be manipulated in a much greater way than analog hearing aids were able to. They allow hearing aids to provide an enhanced sound signal that is more comfortable and allow for clearer speech sounds, especially speech sounds in the high frequencies.

Digital hearing aids also allow Audiologists to make major adjustments to the devices' programs improving the patient's comfort and hearing. When compressing a normal hearing range of 120 decibels, to a reduced hearing range of 20-50 decibels, or providing amplification for a mild hearing loss, digital devices provide a much improved speech signal.

Digital devices allow hearing aids to provide more comfortable, clearer speech sounds, especially in the high frequencies (letter sounds such as s, th, f, sh, ch, p, k and t) which are the most important sounds for understanding speech. Fine tuning adjustments for each frequency are made to better match the needs of patients.

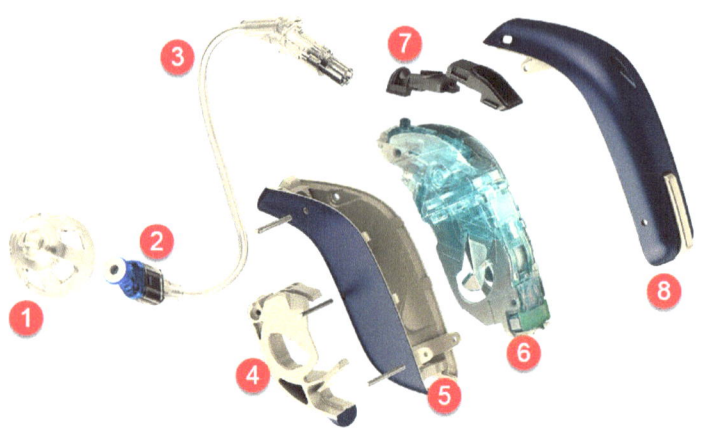

Hearing Device Components

1 – Dome	5 – Hearing aid case
2 – Receiver or Speaker	6 – Amplifier
3 – Receiver wire	7 - Microphones
4 – Battery drawer	8 – Top of case and controls

Hearing aid batteries are required for all hearing aids. Most batteries are changed by the user on a regular basis. Others may use rechargeable batteries.

Because hearing aids are exposed to daily changes in temperature, moisture due to perspiration or an accidental shower with the hearing aid on – hearing aids sometimes stop functioning, or function at reduced levels. Oils from skin, make-up, hairspray, and even dry skin or dirt can get into the nooks and crannies of hearing aids and stop them from operating.

CARING FOR YOUR HEARING AIDS

In order to operate well, hearing devices should be cleaned every day. Yes, I did say every day... Each time you insert the device in your ear, it may pick up ear wax, or other substances that can damage it. The degree to which you need to carefully clean will vary depending on your individual situation. Talk to your hearing care provider to find out the best way to clean your device and supplies to best protect the aids, but general advice for cleaning and care involves:

- **Wipe it down:** At night when you take out your hearing device: wipe with a soft cloth to dry off or polish the hearing aid. Remove wax, dirt, moisture, sunscreen, or make-up that may find its way into the microphone openings, or the sound port.
- **Brush** off any wax that is stuck with a small brush.
- **Look closely:** Examine each hearing aid to see if the sound port and microphones have any debris that should be removed. You may need a magnifier to see these since they are very small.
- **Filters and domes:** Most hearing devices have replaceable filters and/or domes on the part of the device that fits in your ear. They need to be changed periodically.

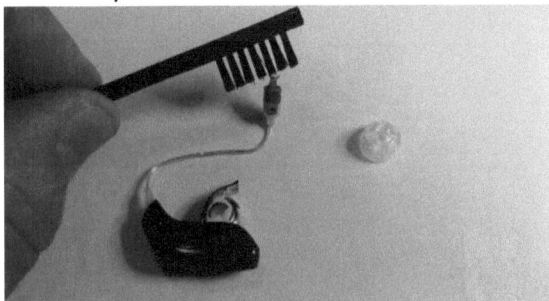

With the dome removed, the speaker can be cleaned with a brush provided with the hearing device

- **Ask your hearing care provider** for cleaning advice for your specific device. They will be very happy to go over the details again and again – since they know that careful cleaning provides better hearing and happier patients!

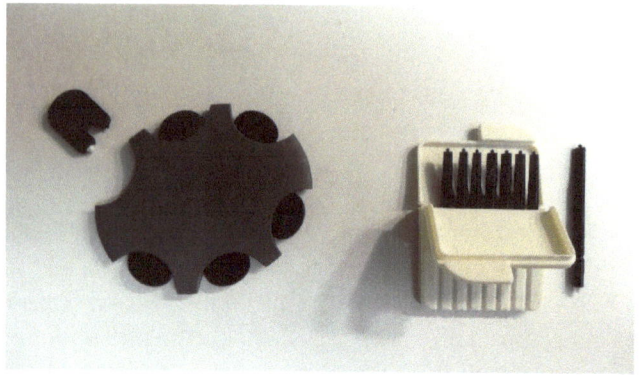

6 – HOW TO CHOOSE AN AUDIOLOGIST

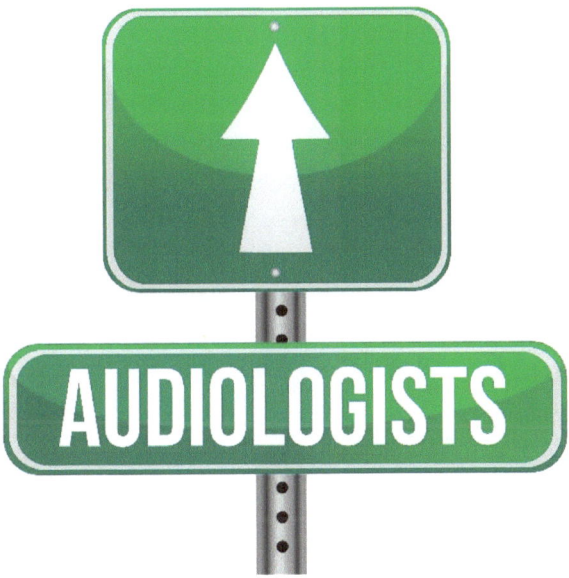

Choosing an audiologist or other hearing care provider is an important decision since you should return to this professional regularly for regular hearing care over a period of many years. You may have discussed this decision with several people before you go to the first appointment. This is a good thing since physicians and experienced hearing aid users may be an excellent resource, often better than any ads you see in the paper or online. When you need your ears evaluated, you may see a few different types of professionals.

Audiologist: For diagnostic hearing evaluations, you will see an audiologist. Using the tools of the hearing evaluation, the audiologist can "see" past your eardrum to determine how your ear is functioning. If there is a medical cause to your hearing loss, the audiologist will know and will refer you to a physician. The audiologist is also able to clean out earwax if needed, and prescribe and fit hearing devices. You are likely to see the same audiologist for many years if you need hearing aids.

Otolaryngologist: Also known as an ENT, this doctor is an expert in the medical causes of hearing loss (as well as noses and throats) and can provide medical treatment or surgery when needed. They can examine your ears generally as far as the eardrum (unless you need surgery) and will also be quite familiar with the hearing evaluation the audiologist performs. Only a few (less than 20%) of hearing losses are medically treatable. When the ENT determines there is no medical cause for your hearing loss, you will be referred back to an audiologist for hearing devices.

Hearing Aid Specialist: Depending on how you start your search for better hearing, you may see a hearing aid specialist. This person is able to do a simplified version of the evaluation done by an audiologist. They are required to refer you to a physician if needed when medical treatment is a possibility. They sell and fit hearing devices.

An audiologist is likely the best person to offer you the most comprehensive advice about your hearing.

If you are looking for an audiologist for the first time, here are five items to consider in meeting your hearing needs.

1: Qualifications

An audiologist is a medical professional specializing in hearing, ear, and balance-related issues. An audiologist's depth of training (master's degree level and beyond) places them in a superior position to a hearing aid dispenser to diagnose and recommend action. This is a bit like the difference between someone buying reading glasses from a pharmacy or visiting the optometrist.

Look for the abbreviations Au.D. (Doctor of Audiology), CCC-A, (Certificate of Clinical Competency in Audiology), MA (Master's Degree in Arts), MS (Master's Degree in Science), HIS (Hearing Instrument Specialist), HAD (Hearing Aid Dispenser), or F-AAA (Fellow of the American Academy of Audiology) after the hearing provider's name as a sign of their professional qualifications.

The Doctor of Audiology who also earned an MA or MS degree is a member of a special group of audiologists who chose to earn a doctorate prior to a requirement to do so. This group usually has more years of experience and education than the person who went straight through to earn the doctorate.

The HIS or HAD is a hearing aid specialist or hearing aid dispenser. At minimum, they have a high school diploma and have received training in hearing aid dispensing. This group of specialists has a state license, but not necessarily any college training in audiology. Many of these specialists are highly dedicated to helping people to hear better, and many work in conjunction with an audiologist.

Types of Hearing Health Care providers	
Doctor of Audiology (has Au.D. & Master's Degree)	The Au.D. title is used, but a Master's degree was earned previously
Doctor of Audiology	Au.D. or Ph.D.
Master's Degree	MA or MS. As of 2007 a doctorate is required for all new Audiologists
Hearing Aid Dispenser	HIS, HAD Minimum high school diploma

2: Care from the audiologist

You will build a long-term relationship with your hearing care provider, as he or she learns about your needs and what does or does not work for you. It is therefore helpful that the clinic plans for you to see the same provider at each visit. Also, consider the attitude of the staff. Are they warm, welcoming and patient, or did you feel rushed or overlooked? How easy is the audiologist to contact after the appointment? You may have questions that occur to you after an appointment. You'll want the opportunity to easily follow up to get your questions answered. Also, inquire if the clinic is able to undertake basic maintenance and minor repairs on site while you wait? This lessens the amount of time you will be without your device if there is a problem. For those times when the device needs to be sent off, do they offer a loaner device?

#3 Brand choice and affiliation

Check that your audiologist is not working for a manufacturer and obligated to any particular brand of hearing aid. This means they can be truly independent when it comes to advice, rather than be influenced by sales requirements.

Also, look to see if they stock a variety of manufacturers' products, since different companies offer different options that you may want for your hearing devices.

4: Payment plans

There's no denying that good quality hearing devices are a financial investment. It is important to purchase the best device you can afford and this may mean spreading out the payments. If this is a service you could make use of, then inquire if this is something the office can arrange. If you have health insurance that covers hearing devices, ask if the office is able to help process the claim for you.

#5 Rapport with the audiologist

This is probably the **most important** detail about finding a new hearing care professional. Find a provider who you can talk to, who will listen to you, and make you feel comfortable. These are some of the most vital features, regardless of other requirements.

Finding the Best Hearing Health Care:

- Speak to friends and relatives
- Ask people who have hearing aids who they see
- Consult a trusted physician
- Visit more than one local audiology office

Websites – These sites may help you to learn more. Keep in mind that some sites charge the audiologist to be listed on the site, so they may not be listed on every site.

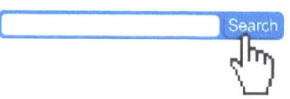

- www.yelp.com
  Read the reviews for local audiologists
- www.Google.com
  Note: The biggest ad is not always the best provider
- www.earq.com
- www.oticon.com
- http://www.audiology.org
- http://hearinghealthfoundation.org
- www.hearingloss.org - The Hearing Loss Association of America
- www.starkey.com
- www.Phonak.com
- www.widex.com
- www.bestsoundtechnology.com – Siemens hearing aids
- www.Cochlear.com

7 - GETTING USED TO HEARING DEVICES

A FREE TRIAL PERIOD

Once the selection of a hearing aid is made, a demonstration model is fit and a trial period begins. Sometimes we have chosen the device that is the best at the beginning of this process. Other times, we try a few different styles or models (like your physician may do with medication) to find one what is the best solution for you. This is a critical step in the fitting process, especially for many patients with a more complex hearing loss. If we rush to fit one device without appropriate evaluation, we could deprive the patient of the best possible outcome. **No matter how much technology or how much the cost, the best hearing aid solution for any patient is the one that will consistently be used. Hearing aids are not effective when they sit in a drawer.**

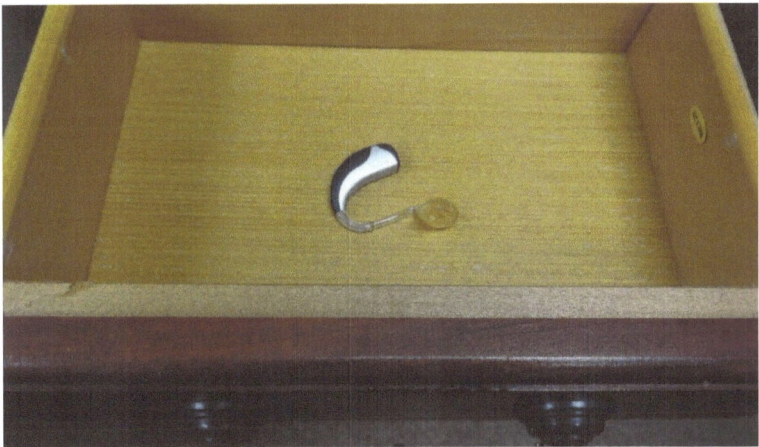

California State requirements (some other states also) allow a FREE 45-day trial period that includes no obligation. This trial period has an important purpose. The typical person takes at least 30 days to adapt to wearing a hearing device. Many people have spent years gradually losing hearing to the degree that when they are fit with hearing aids, they hear quite a few sounds that they do not recognize. Paper rustling, background noise, water running, and frequently the sound of the person's voice are foreign sounds that the individual wearing the hearing aid does not recognize. Someone new to wearing hearing aids needs to adjust to hearing all these sounds again.

This period of adjustment is vital to success with hearing aids. Learning how to use the devices and clean them as needed is difficult for some people. Regular use during the trial period is very important since there are so many sounds that a person hears that they need to identify. It takes time operating the devices to understand how they work to help you hear. Often, adjustments to the hearing aids by your hearing care provider are made to make sound more comfortable. All this helps patients acclimate to wearing the devices.

Keep track of your responses to sounds you hear around you as you adjust to your new hearing aids and discuss with your audiologist. Are there sounds that are too loud or annoying? Are there noises you feel you will get used to, but are new to you? Are there sounds you have not heard in years and are happy to hear them again?

Because it is a no obligation trial period, there are some people who will try hearing aids, and then return them during the 45 day period. Perhaps they realize that they are not ready to wear hearing devices. Maybe finances are an issue. Sometimes, a significant other is not supportive in the trial period with hearing devices. At this point, we discuss the reasons, and make a plan for future follow up when the patient feels they may be ready to continue this process. All hearing aids that are fit in California are fit by this schedule – the time frame and the ability to change one's mind is an important protection for the hearing impaired consumer.

Things to do during your 45 Day Trial Checklist	
	Wear your new hearing aids as often as possible
	Go to the places you usually go such as stores or work, and also places you go less frequently
	Make sure you are mostly comfortable – bring a hearing aid holder with you in case things are too loud and you have to remove the hearing aids and store them
	If you have hearing aid controls, turn the hearing aids up or down if you need to
	Make lists for your audiologist – sounds you hear that you like, and sounds that bother you. This will help your provider adjust your hearing aids
	Clean your hearing aids every day to avoid earwax blocking the sound
	Call your audiologist for an earlier follow up appointment if you need to – especially if you are uncomfortable or feel like you do not want to wear the hearing aids
	If you think you may want to try a different model of hearing aid, contact the audiologist a few days before so they can order a different style for you before the appointment
	Please make notes below on other activities and what you did or did not like about your hearing devices

8 – ABOUT THE AUTHOR

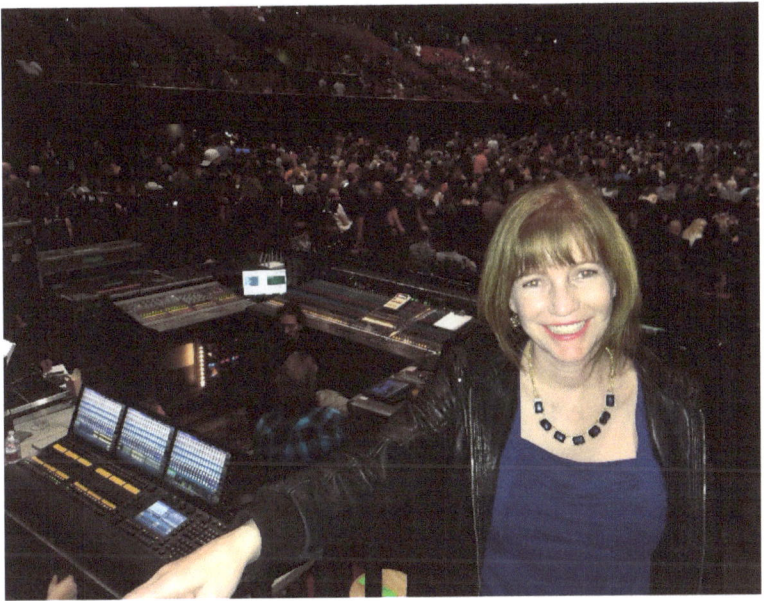

I've always been drawn to sound and hearing. Here I am at a concert - checking out the control booth. As you may have guessed, I remembered to wear my music earplugs during the concert to protect my ears.

A Note from the Author

After growing up in a household with a father with a severe hearing loss, and a mother who did not understand hearing problems, I have always wanted to help those with auditory challenges. I spent my time in college and university exploring different topics related to people with special needs, but discovered audiology finally. After an initial career as a teacher, and some time raising children, I found a career that I had a passion for. You might say that I've been obsessed with hearing for the last 20 plus years. Everywhere I go, I'm always talking to people about their hearing and how to improve or protect it. I've been known to pass out ear plugs to construction workers I pass on the street or reach into someone's ear to adjust a hearing aid that I notice is not in straight while I am at the market.

If you live in my area of Southern California, I'd love to see you in my office, but if that's not possible, I'd still like to help you.

Please feel free to email me at HearingHealthAdvice@yahoo.com if you have any questions or would like any advice on how you can hear better!

About the Author

Patrice Rifkind has lived in the Santa Clarita Valley for over 30 years. As a resident of the SCV, Patrice and her husband Ken raised three children that are grown and have advanced degrees. Patrice aspired to become an audiologist at the age of 20, beginning her career as a special education teacher. Her desire to help her father and other people later motivated her to attain a Master's degree and Doctorate degree in audiology.

Patrice has been an owner of Audiology Associates Hearing Center in the Santa Clarita Valley for over 15 years where she helps people hear better and communicate with their friends, family, and coworkers. Patrice has personally treated thousands of patients in the Santa Clarita Valley. She has often provided low cost or free hearing devices to people who could not afford them. She is an outspoken advocate for hearing health care and often speaks publicly to educate the community on how to protect their hearing. Audiology Associates gives away several hundred sets of ear plugs each year towards this goal at gun tournaments and music festivals.

Dr. Rifkind is an active member of Zonta, Assistance League, and the SCV Senior Resource Alliance. She likes to attend community events such as the Celebrity Waiter, Boys' and Girls' Club Auction, Lunafest, Sunset on the Vineyard, Sip and Stroll, SCV Jazz Festival, as a volunteer or as an attendee.

Testimonials from a few of the people that I have worked with:

I had an industrial accident and now need hearing aids. I have been to three audiologists in the past per workers' compensation rules. This Office, above all others, is by far the best. I was treated by Dr. Patrice Rifkind who spent roughly 2 hours with me explaining how hearing aids work and teaching me all the intricate parts, and answered all my questions. These doctors truly care about their patients I would highly recommend going here for hearing aids.   Bret R - Santa Clarita

My name is Pete and I'm a longtime patient of Patrice (Patti) Rifkind and Audiology Associates. Because of the outstanding care and service I've received here, I feel it necessary to share my experience with others.

What many people don't know is that there's a big difference between a hearing aid dispenser and a highly trained and experienced audiologist professional. If you've ever been told you might need a hearing aid, I suggest going over to Audiology Associates because you can be assured you will see a highly trained and qualified professional and receive the best care.

If you need a hearing aid, you will be surprised at how much better you can hear when you get your aid. For those with hearing problems, a great audiologist like Patti, and a good hearing aid, can make a major positive impact on your life!
Pete G – Santa Clarita

The Audiology Associates team are the best. Dr. Patrice Rifkind really takes her time to understand her patient's needs and provides the BEST service and results you can ask for. I can't say enough about the courteous and accommodating staff she has. My entire family sees her and I would highly recommend them to everyone! Thank you Patrice!   Mike T - Valencia

I have been going to Patrice for 16 years. I was 47 when I met her and I thought I was too young to wear hearing aids. I was so wrong. Patrice has changed my life for the better. She sets the tone for what your experience is going to be like. Patrice is not only patient, but she is so well educated in her field that I know that she can listen to what problems I am having and solve them. I feel blessed to have found Patrice Rifkind and Audiology Associates - and will always use them and recommend.
Joel V - Santa Clarita

I'm a 59 year old business guy who relies on senses to navigate through daily situations, I'm also a grandfather who was missing a lot. Also getting older and a bit worried about perception people have of the old guy wearing hearing aids.
I've had hearing loss my whole life. I've been to audiologist but never did anything, even had unsuccessful surgery to improve my hearing, but then just learned to live with it.
On an impulse I went in to Audiologist Assoc. looking for the in ear canal aid that no one can see, but then Patrice guided me through the realization quality hearing is more important than vanity. My wife and I learned a lot about my poor hearing and its impact on our quality of life. I went home with a trial set thinking I might as well see what it's like, but would never actually keep them.
The next day I was outside and heard our five year old neighbor boy talking, and I actually understood what he was saying. I always talked to Ty, but honestly never really got what he was talking about. Pretty sad, I was missing the world through a smart young kids words.
Been a month now and I just bought the hearing aids from Patrice. I honestly no longer care who notices. I know my coworkers appreciate me no longer saying, "What?" I really enjoy my 16 month old twin grandkids talking to me. They don't really talk yet, but I seem to understand, the sounds are magic. Oh, and my wife likes the fact our TV is no longer blasting.

If you don't hear well, go see Patrice. There are few true caring professionals in healthcare today, it's tough to give patients time and make money, but my wife and I got all the time we needed. Patrice is a true caring pro! Life is too short to miss hearing birds, wind, dogs barking, and the sound of a well hit tennis ball. Go see Patrice and get her help, you will enjoy life a little more. Simple. Do it. Thank you Patrice!!

Tim A - Santa Clarita

Tim, you got lucky. On a whim you went to see an audiologist but you were seen and helped by THE BEST AUDIOLOGIST! She invests herself completely in her clients improved living through better hearing. Welcome to the fan club.

Len C - Santa Clarita

And from a colleague:

I have had the pleasure of knowing Dr. Patrice Rifkind, both personally and professionally for the past 20 years. Dr. Rifkind has always stood out for her work ethic, her dedication to her profession, her treatment of her patients and management of her business and her associates. As a fellow audiologist and business associate, I have always admired how Dr. Rifkind handles the running of her business and the empathy she shows all her patients. I have spoken to other professionals in the field and it appears they all have the same high regard for Dr. Rifkind. It is no wonder that her business continues to grow throughout the years. I certainly have no hesitancy in recommending Dr. Rifkind for any hearing health care needs.

Gary Dorf, Au.D.
Audiologist

Acknowledgements

Thank you!

My heartfelt thanks to Joel and Cydney Fox for their amazing contributions, guidance, and friendship. Also Joel for your expert writing advice. Thank you so much Ken for being my project manager for this book, and an all-around terrific husband. I appreciate the family of Audiology Associates: Dr. Kevin, Dede, Linda, Brando, Cheryl, Haley, Kimberly and Celeste who help me to help others. Last, but not least – thank you to my patients who have taught me much about life, and allow me to teach them and help them hear better. I LOVE MY JOB!

Photos and images

Thank you very much to our photographers for all of the photos and images in this book. Photos were provided by Brian and Lindsay Schlick of Schlick Art, Circe Denyer and by Ken Rifkind. Other images provided by Oticon Inc. and Stock images licensed by Shutterstock.

www.ingramcontent.com/pod-product-compliance
Lightning Source LLC
Chambersburg PA
CBHW050812290526
45792CB00001B/82